Adaptogens Guide for Beginners

Creating an Adaptogenic Wellness Plan

By

Raghnall Alfred

Copyright@2023

Table of Contents

CHAPTER 1 7

Introduction..............................7

1.1 What are Adaptogens 7

1.2 How Do Adaptogens Work

....9

1.3 Benefits of Using

Adaptogens.............................11

CHAPTER 2 14

Getting Started with Adaptogens

....14

2.1 Assessing Your Wellness

Goals 14

2.2 Consultation with a

Healthcare Professional.........16

2.3 Types of Adaptogens and

Their Uses 18

CHAPTER 3 22

Popular Adaptogens and Their Properties 22

3.1 Ashwagandha (Withania somnifera) 22

3.2 Rhodiola Rosea 23

3.3 Holy Basil (Tulsi)............24

3.4 Ginseng 25

3.5 Eleuthero (Siberian Ginseng) 26

3.6 Adaptogenic Blends 26

CHAPTER 4 29

Incorporating Adaptogens into Your Routine 29

4.1 Choosing the Right Form: Capsules, Powders, Teas, etc. 30

4.2 Proper Dosage Guidelines 34

4.3 When to Take Adaptogens: Morning or Night? 37

4.4 Mixing Adaptogens with Other Supplements.................39

CHAPTER 5 45

Potential Considerations and Precautions..............................45

5.1 Possible Interactions with Medications............................46

5.2 Allergic Reactions and Side Effects 48

5.3 Notable Groups Who Should Avoid Adaptogens 50

CHAPTER 6 56

Lifestyle Factors and Adaptogen Synergy 56

6.1 Diet and Nutrition 56

6.2 Sleep and Stress Management.......................58

6.3 Physical Activity and Exercise....................61

6.4 Mindfulness and Meditation 62

CHAPTER 7 65

Creating an Adaptogenic Wellness Plan.......................65

7.1 Personalizing Your Adaptogen Regimen..............65

7.2 Tracking Progress and Adjustments 70

7.3 Long-Term Benefits and Sustainable Practices.............74

CHAPTER 8 79

Recipes and DIY Adaptogen
Creations 79

8.1 Adaptogenic Smoothie
Recipes 79

8.2 Herbal Tea Blends...........85

8.3 Incorporating Adaptogens
into Meals...................................89

CHAPTER 1

Introduction

In our fast-paced and often stressful modern lives, maintaining a healthy balance is essential for overall well-being. This is where adaptogens come into play, offering a natural and holistic approach to supporting our bodies' ability to adapt to stressors.

1.1 What are Adaptogens

Adaptogens are a class of natural substances, predominantly plant-derived, that have gained significant attention for their unique ability to help the body resist and adapt to various stressors, be they physical, emotional, or environmental. These stressors can range from the demands of a high-pressure job to the challenges of daily life, and even include exposure to pollutants and toxins. What sets adaptogens apart is their capacity to modulate the body's stress response system, bringing it back into balance when it becomes overwhelmed.

Adaptogens work by interacting with a complex network of bodily systems, including the hypothalamic-pituitary-adrenal (HPA) axis and the sympathetic nervous system. These systems play pivotal roles in managing stress and maintaining homeostasis. Unlike conventional medications, which tend to force specific physiological responses, adaptogens exhibit a bidirectional effect, meaning they can both stimulate and calm these systems as needed. This adaptogenic response is why they are revered for their ability to provide energy when fatigued or to promote relaxation when anxious.

1.2 How Do Adaptogens Work

The intricate mechanisms through which adaptogens work involve a series of interconnected pathways that regulate stress and energy levels within the body. One of the primary mechanisms involves the modulation of cortisol, often referred to as the "stress hormone." Adaptogens help regulate cortisol production, preventing it from becoming excessively high during times of stress or too low when energy is needed. By fine-tuning cortisol levels, adaptogens aid in preventing the detrimental effects of chronic stress, such as adrenal fatigue and compromised immune function.

Moreover, adaptogens engage with the body's cellular stress response system. This involves activating proteins and pathways that bolster cellular resilience and repair, thereby enhancing the body's ability to withstand a variety of stressors. Adaptogens also work to maintain balanced levels of neurotransmitters, the chemical messengers that play a critical role in mood regulation, cognitive function, and emotional well-being.

1.3 Benefits of Using Adaptogens

The benefits of incorporating adaptogens into your lifestyle are wide-ranging and can positively impact various facets of your physical and mental well-being. Some key benefits include:

- **Stress Resilience:** Adaptogens are renowned for their stress-reducing properties. They assist the body in responding to stress more efficiently, helping to prevent burnout and fatigue.

- **Energy and Vitality:** By regulating energy levels, adaptogens can provide a sustained boost in vitality without the jitters associated with stimulants.

- **Cognitive Function:** Adaptogens support cognitive health by enhancing mental clarity, focus, and memory.

- **Immune Support:** Many adaptogens possess immune-modulating properties, aiding the immune system in staying robust and responsive.

- **Hormonal Balance:** Adaptogens can help regulate hormone production, making them particularly beneficial for individuals dealing with hormonal imbalances.

- **Emotional Well-being:** Adaptogens can promote a sense of calm and relaxation, which can be particularly helpful for managing anxiety and promoting emotional balance.

In essence, adaptogens offer a holistic approach to wellness by promoting harmony between the mind and body. As you delve into the world of adaptogens, it's important to remember that their effects are gradual and often cumulative. It's not about instant results, but rather a commitment to a healthier and more balanced lifestyle.

CHAPTER 2

Getting Started with Adaptogens

Navigating the world of adaptogens can be an exciting and rewarding journey toward better well-being. However, it's important to approach this journey with careful consideration and proper guidance.

2.1 Assessing Your Wellness Goals

Before incorporating adaptogens into your routine, take the time to reflect on your wellness goals and objectives. Are you seeking stress relief, improved energy levels, better sleep, enhanced cognitive function, or a combination of these benefits? Understanding your intentions will help you choose the most appropriate adaptogens to support your specific needs.

Consider creating a list of your primary wellness goals and any secondary objectives you'd like to address. For example, if stress reduction is your main goal, you might want to focus on adaptogens known for their calming properties. On the other hand, if you're aiming to boost energy and vitality, adaptogens with energizing effects might be more suitable.

2.2 Consultation with a Healthcare Professional

While adaptogens are generally considered safe for most people, it's always wise to consult a healthcare professional before making any significant changes to your wellness routine, especially if you have pre-existing health conditions, take medications, are pregnant, or are breastfeeding.

A healthcare professional, such as a doctor, naturopath, or registered dietitian, can provide personalized guidance based on your individual health history, medications, and specific needs. They can help you identify any potential interactions between adaptogens and medications you're taking, as well as ensure that your chosen adaptogens align with your overall health goals.

During your consultation, be sure to provide a comprehensive overview of your health status, including any known allergies, medical conditions, or medications. This information will allow the healthcare professional to make informed recommendations tailored to your situation.

By collaborating with a healthcare professional, you'll receive evidence-based advice on adaptogen selection, dosages, and potential interactions, ultimately ensuring that your journey with adaptogens is safe and effective.

The goal of incorporating adaptogens into your routine is to enhance your well-being and support your body's natural resilience. With careful consideration of your goals and expert guidance, you'll be well-equipped to embark on a successful and beneficial adaptogen experience.

2.3 Types of Adaptogens and Their Uses

In your journey to explore the world of adaptogens, it's essential to become familiar with the various types of adaptogenic herbs and their specific uses. Each adaptogen offers a unique set of benefits, making it important to select the ones that align with your wellness goals. Here, we'll introduce you to some common adaptogens and their associated uses:

1. **Ashwagandha (Withania somnifera):**

- **Uses:** Ashwagandha is renowned for its stress-relieving properties. It helps balance cortisol levels, promoting a calm and focused mind. It's also used to enhance energy and support the nervous system.

2. **Rhodiola Rosea:**

- **Uses:** Rhodiola is often chosen for its energy-boosting and mood-enhancing effects. It can help combat fatigue, improve cognitive function, and increase resilience to stress.

3. **Holy Basil (Tulsi):**

- **Uses:** Holy Basil is prized for its adaptogenic and calming qualities. It supports the body's response to stress, aids in relaxation, and may contribute to improved sleep quality.

4. **Ginseng (Panax ginseng and others):**

- **Uses:** Ginseng is known for its vitality-enhancing properties. It can improve energy levels, cognitive function, and physical endurance. Different types of ginseng, such as Asian and American ginseng, offer varying benefits.

5. **Eleuthero (Siberian Ginseng):**

- **Uses:** Eleuthero is used to boost stamina and resilience. It supports the body's ability to adapt to stressors, making it a popular choice for enhancing overall vitality.

6. **Adaptogenic Blends:**

- **Uses:** These blends combine various adaptogens to create synergistic effects. They are often formulated to provide a broad spectrum of benefits, such as stress reduction, improved cognitive function, and enhanced immune support.

When selecting adaptogens, it's important to consider both your primary wellness goals and any secondary benefits you're seeking. For example, if you're aiming to manage stress and also need an energy boost, a combination of ashwagandha and rhodiola might be beneficial.

Moreover, pay attention to the form in which adaptogens are available, such as capsules, powders, teas, or tinctures. Each form has its advantages, and you can choose based on your preferences and lifestyle.

As you explore adaptogens, keep in mind that individual responses can vary. What works well for one person might not have the same effects for another. Start with a single adaptogen and observe how your body responds before introducing multiple adaptogens at once.

CHAPTER 3

Popular Adaptogens and Their Properties

we'll explore some of the most popular adaptogens and their unique properties. Each of these adaptogens offers distinct benefits for stress management, energy enhancement, cognitive function, and overall well-being. Let's delve into the details:

3.1 Ashwagandha (Withania somnifera)

- **Properties:** Ashwagandha, also known as "Indian ginseng," is celebrated for its adaptogenic and calming properties. It helps regulate cortisol levels, promoting a balanced stress response. It's known to reduce anxiety, improve sleep quality, and enhance cognitive function.

- **Uses:** Ashwagandha is often used to alleviate stress-related symptoms, boost resilience to stress, and support relaxation. It's also utilized for improving energy levels, cognitive performance, and overall vitality.

3.2 Rhodiola Rosea

- **Properties:** Rhodiola is valued for its energy-boosting and mood-enhancing effects. It enhances the body's ability to adapt to physical and emotional stressors. It's believed to increase mental clarity, focus, and alertness.

- **Uses:** Rhodiola is commonly used to combat fatigue, reduce feelings of burnout, and enhance physical and mental endurance. It's also sought after for its potential to improve mood and alleviate symptoms of depression.

3.3 Holy Basil (Tulsi)

- **Properties:** Holy Basil, also known as Tulsi, is revered for its adaptogenic and calming qualities. It's rich in antioxidants and supports the body's response to stress, helping to restore balance to the nervous system.

- **Uses:** Holy Basil is used to reduce stress, anxiety, and inflammation. It's also known to promote relaxation, enhance mental clarity,

and support overall emotional
well-being.

3.4 Ginseng

- **Properties:** Ginseng, available in various forms such as Asian and American ginseng, is prized for its vitality-enhancing effects. It boosts energy levels, enhances cognitive function, and improves physical endurance.

- **Uses:** Ginseng is used to increase stamina, reduce fatigue, and improve overall energy levels. It's also believed to support immune function and hormonal balance.

3.5 Eleuthero (Siberian Ginseng)

- **Properties:** Eleuthero, also known as Siberian ginseng, is known for its adaptogenic and immune-supportive properties. It helps the body cope with stress, enhance endurance, and strengthen resilience.

- **Uses:** Eleuthero is commonly used to increase physical and mental stamina, especially during times of stress or high activity. It's also sought after for its potential to support overall immune system function.

3.6 Adaptogenic Blends

- **Properties:** Adaptogenic blends combine various adaptogens to create synergistic effects. These blends are often formulated to provide a comprehensive range of benefits, targeting stress reduction, energy enhancement, and cognitive support.

- **Uses:** Adaptogenic blends are versatile and can address multiple wellness goals simultaneously. They're a convenient option for those seeking a balanced combination of adaptogenic effects.

As you explore these popular adaptogens, consider your specific wellness goals and consult with a healthcare professional to determine which ones align with your needs. Keep in mind that individual responses can vary, so it's important to start with a lower dose and gradually increase as needed.

Incorporating adaptogens into your daily routine can contribute to a more resilient and balanced lifestyle.

CHAPTER 4

Incorporating Adaptogens into Your Routine

Embracing adaptogens into your daily routine can be a transformative step toward better well-being. However, the form in which you choose to consume adaptogens can significantly impact your experience. Here we'll explore the various forms of adaptogens available and offer insights into choosing the right one for you.

4.1 Choosing the Right Form: Capsules, Powders, Teas, etc.

Adaptogens come in different forms, each with its own advantages and considerations. Selecting the form that suits your preferences and lifestyle can enhance your overall adaptogen experience. Here are some common forms of adaptogens and their features:

1. **Capsules or Tablets:**

- **Advantages:** Capsules and tablets provide a convenient and standardized dosage. They are easy to incorporate into your daily routine and are often tasteless, making them ideal for those who prefer simplicity.

- **Considerations:** Some capsules may contain additional ingredients as binders or fillers. Read the ingredient list carefully if you have dietary restrictions or sensitivities.

2. **Powders:**

- **Advantages:** Powders allow for flexibility in dosing and can be easily mixed into smoothies, yogurt, or beverages. This form gives you control over the amount you consume.

- **Considerations:** The taste of certain adaptogenic powders might be strong or bitter. Mixing them into flavored foods or drinks can help mask the taste.

3. **Teas and Infusions:**

- **Advantages:** Adaptogenic teas offer a soothing way to consume these herbs. They can promote relaxation and stress relief, making them a great option for winding down.

- **Considerations:** The concentration of adaptogenic compounds in teas might be lower compared to capsules or powders. Steeping times and water temperature can affect the potency of the tea.

4. **Tinctures:**

- **Advantages:** Tinctures are liquid extracts that provide a concentrated form of adaptogens. They offer rapid absorption and can be taken sublingually (under the tongue).

- **Considerations:** Tinctures often have an alcohol base, which might not be suitable for everyone. Some individuals may find the taste strong or bitter.

5. **Adaptogenic Blends:**

- **Advantages:** Blends combine multiple adaptogens in one product, offering a diverse range of benefits. They are designed to deliver a balanced combination of effects.

- **Considerations:** Blends might contain a smaller quantity of each adaptogen compared to standalone products. Be sure to choose a blend that aligns with your wellness goals.

When choosing the right form, consider your lifestyle, taste preferences, and how easily you can incorporate adaptogens into your routine. It's also important to start with a lower dose and gradually increase as needed. Keep in mind that consistency is key—adaptogens work best when taken regularly over time.

Before making a decision, consult with a healthcare professional to ensure that the chosen form of adaptogens is safe and appropriate for your individual health needs. With the right form in hand, you'll be well on your way to reaping the benefits of these remarkable natural remedies.

4.2 Proper Dosage Guidelines

Incorporating adaptogens into your daily routine can be a transformative step toward better well-being. However, the timing and dosage of adaptogen consumption are crucial for optimal results.

Determining the right dosage of adaptogens can vary based on factors such as the specific adaptogen, your individual needs, and the form you're using. It's essential to start with a lower dose and gradually increase as your body adjusts. Here are some general dosage guidelines:

- **Capsules or Tablets:** Follow the manufacturer's recommended dosage on the packaging. This is usually a standardized dose that simplifies dosing.

- **Powders:** Start with a small amount, typically around 1/4 to 1/2 teaspoon, and gradually increase every few days as needed. You can mix the powder into water, smoothies, yogurt, or other foods.

- **Teas and Infusions:** Brew adaptogenic teas according to the instructions provided. You might need to steep them a bit longer than regular teas to extract the beneficial compounds.

- **Tinctures:** Follow the recommended dosage on the tincture bottle. Tinctures are often concentrated, so a few drops can be sufficient.

- **Adaptogenic Blends:** Adhere to the recommended dosage on the product label. Blends are formulated to provide a balanced combination of adaptogens, so following the suggested serving size is crucial.

Individual responses can vary, so what works for one person might differ for another. Listen to your body and pay attention to how you feel after taking adaptogens. If you experience any adverse effects, consult a healthcare professional.

4.3 When to Take Adaptogens: Morning or Night?

The timing of adaptogen consumption can influence their effects on your body's energy levels and stress response. Here are some considerations for deciding when to take adaptogens:

- **Morning:** Many adaptogens, such as rhodiola and ginseng, have energizing effects and can support focus and vitality. Taking them in the morning can help you start your day on a positive note.

- **Midday:** If you experience an energy slump in the afternoon, taking adaptogens around midday can help you maintain focus and stamina throughout the day.

- **Evening:** Some adaptogens, like ashwagandha and holy basil, have calming properties that can support relaxation and better sleep. Taking them in the evening can help you unwind and prepare for restful sleep.

- **Twice a Day:** Depending on your needs, you might choose to take adaptogens both in the morning and evening. For example, you could take energizing adaptogens in the morning and calming ones in the evening.

Ultimately, the best time to take adaptogens depends on your individual schedule and desired outcomes. Pay attention to how different adaptogens affect you and adjust your timing accordingly. Remember that consistency is key—regular use over time is more likely to yield noticeable benefits.

As always, consult with a healthcare professional before making changes to your supplement routine, especially if you're taking medications or have underlying health conditions. Their guidance can help you make informed decisions about dosing and timing based on your unique needs.

4.4 Mixing Adaptogens with Other Supplements

Integrating adaptogens into your daily routine can be a transformative step toward improved well-being. If you're already taking other supplements, you might be wondering about the compatibility of adaptogens with your current regimen.

Combining adaptogens with other supplements is a common practice, and it can often be done safely and effectively. However, it's important to approach this combination with caution and awareness. Here are some factors to consider:

1. **Consult with a Healthcare Professional:** Before introducing new supplements, including adaptogens, into your routine, consult with a healthcare professional. They can provide personalized advice based on your health history, medications, and specific needs.

2. **Research Potential Interactions:**
    Some adaptogens and supplements
    can interact with each other or
    with medications you're taking.
    For example, adaptogens with
    potential blood-thinning effects
    might interact with anticoagulant
    medications. Do your research or
    consult a healthcare professional to
    identify any potential interactions.

3. **Start Slowly:** If you're introducing
    multiple supplements at once,
    consider starting with one at a
    time. This will help you monitor
    your body's response and identify
    any adverse effects or interactions.

4. **Dosage Adjustments:** If you're
    taking adaptogens in addition to
    other supplements, you might need
    to adjust the dosages of each to
    ensure you're not exceeding

recommended limits for specific nutrients or compounds.

5. **Monitor Your Body:** Pay close attention to how your body responds to the combination of supplements. If you experience any unusual symptoms or discomfort, consult a healthcare professional.

6. **Natural Synergy:** Some adaptogens and supplements have synergistic effects, meaning they can enhance each other's benefits. For example, combining an adaptogen that supports cognitive function with omega-3 fatty acids might have a positive impact on brain health.

7. **Quality Matters:** Choose high-quality supplements from reputable sources. Poor-quality

supplements might contain fillers, contaminants, or inconsistent dosages.

8. **Keep Records:** Maintain a record of the supplements you're taking, including dosages and timing. This will be helpful when discussing your regimen with healthcare professionals.

Individual responses to supplements can vary. What works well for one person might not have the same effects for another. It's important to prioritize your safety and well-being by seeking expert advice and staying informed about the supplements you're taking.

As you explore combining adaptogens with other supplements, remember that a balanced and varied diet is a crucial foundation for overall health.

Supplements should complement a healthy lifestyle rather than replace it. With the right approach, you can create a well-rounded supplement regimen that supports your wellness goals.

CHAPTER 5

Potential Considerations and Precautions

While adaptogens offer numerous benefits for well-being, it's important to approach their usage with careful consideration and awareness of potential interactions and reactions. we'll discuss key considerations and precautions to keep in mind when incorporating adaptogens into your routine.

5.1 Possible Interactions with Medications

Interactions between adaptogens and medications are possible, and it's crucial to be mindful of these interactions to ensure your safety and well-being. Here's what you should consider:

- **Consult with a Healthcare Professional:** Before starting any new supplements, including adaptogens, consult with your healthcare provider, especially if you're taking prescription medications. Some adaptogens can interact with medications and alter their effects.

- **Anticoagulant Medications:** Certain adaptogens, such as ginkgo biloba and garlic, can have anticoagulant effects. If you're on blood-thinning medications, these interactions can lead to increased bleeding risk.

- **Blood Sugar Regulation:** Some adaptogens, like ginseng, may affect blood sugar levels. If you're taking medications for diabetes or blood sugar regulation, adaptogens could impact your medication's effectiveness.

- **Blood Pressure Medications:** Adaptogens with potential effects on blood pressure, such as licorice root and certain ginseng varieties, could interact with blood pressure medications.

- **Thyroid Conditions:** Certain adaptogens, like ashwagandha, may influence thyroid function. If you have thyroid issues and are taking thyroid medications, consult a healthcare professional before using adaptogens.

5.2 Allergic Reactions and Side Effects

Adaptogens are generally well-tolerated, but some individuals might experience allergic reactions or side effects. Here's what to be aware of:

- **Allergic Reactions:** Some adaptogens are part of plant families that could trigger allergic reactions in individuals with known sensitivities. If you have plant allergies, research the adaptogen's botanical family and consult a healthcare professional before use.

- **Gastrointestinal Upset:** In some cases, adaptogens might cause gastrointestinal discomfort, such as upset stomach or diarrhea. Start with a lower dose to assess your tolerance.

- **Stimulating Effects:** Adaptogens like ginseng and rhodiola can have stimulating effects. Taking them too close to bedtime might interfere with sleep. Opt for calming adaptogens in the evening.

- **Individual Variability:** Individual responses to adaptogens can vary. What works well for one person might cause discomfort or adverse effects in another.

- **Pregnancy and Breastfeeding:** Pregnant or breastfeeding individuals should exercise caution when using adaptogens. Some adaptogens are contraindicated during pregnancy due to their

potential impact on hormone
levels.

While adaptogens can offer valuable
support for your well-being, their
usage should be guided by thorough
research, consultation with healthcare
professionals, and awareness of
potential interactions and side effects.
It's always better to err on the side of
caution and prioritize your health and
safety. By being informed and
cautious, you can harness the benefits
of adaptogens while minimizing
potential risks.

5.3 Notable Groups Who Should Avoid Adaptogens

While adaptogens can offer a range of benefits for many individuals, there are certain groups who should exercise caution or avoid their use altogether. Here's a look at notable groups that might need to avoid or limit their use of adaptogens:

1. **Pregnant and Breastfeeding Individuals:**

- **Consideration:** Pregnancy and breastfeeding are critical periods when the body's hormonal balance is already undergoing significant changes. Some adaptogens, especially those that affect hormone levels, might not be suitable during these phases.

2. **Children and Adolescents:**

- **Consideration:** Limited research is available on the safety and effectiveness of adaptogen use in children and adolescents. Their developing bodies might respond differently to adaptogens, so it's best to consult a healthcare professional before considering their use.

3. **Individuals with Autoimmune Conditions:**

- **Consideration:** Adaptogens can influence the immune system, which might pose risks for individuals with autoimmune disorders. Certain adaptogens might trigger immune responses that could worsen autoimmune symptoms.

4. **People Undergoing Surgery:**

- **Consideration:** Some adaptogens can affect blood clotting or blood pressure. If you're scheduled for surgery, it's advisable to discontinue adaptogen use beforehand to minimize the risk of complications during the surgical procedure.

5. **Individuals on Blood-Thinning Medications:**

- **Consideration:** Adaptogens like ginkgo biloba and garlic can have anticoagulant effects, potentially interacting with blood-thinning medications and increasing the risk of bleeding. Consult with a healthcare professional before using adaptogens.

6. **Those with Hormone-Sensitive Conditions:**

- **Consideration:** Adaptogens that influence hormone levels, such as licorice root and some ginseng varieties, might not be suitable for individuals with hormone-sensitive conditions like breast cancer.

7. **Individuals with Specific Allergies:**

- **Consideration:** Some adaptogens belong to botanical families that could trigger allergic reactions in individuals with sensitivities to those families. It's important to research and consult a healthcare professional if you have known allergies.

8. **People with Severe Health Conditions:**

- **Consideration:** Individuals with severe health conditions, particularly those under the care of healthcare professionals, should consult their doctors before introducing adaptogens. Their conditions and medications might interact with adaptogens.

If you fall into any of these groups or have underlying health concerns, it's crucial to consult a healthcare professional before considering adaptogen use. They can provide personalized guidance based on your specific circumstances, ensuring your safety and well-being. While adaptogens can offer numerous benefits for many individuals, the priority should always be your health and the guidance of medical professionals.

CHAPTER 6

Lifestyle Factors and Adaptogen Synergy

The effectiveness of adaptogens isn't solely dependent on their consumption; your overall lifestyle plays a significant role in maximizing their benefits. we'll explore two critical lifestyle factors that synergize with adaptogen use: diet and nutrition, as well as sleep and stress management.

6.1 Diet and Nutrition

The foods you consume can impact how well your body responds to adaptogens. A balanced and nourishing diet provides a solid foundation for adaptogen synergy. Consider the following:

- **Whole Foods:** Prioritize a diet rich in whole, unprocessed foods. Fruits, vegetables, lean proteins, whole grains, and healthy fats provide essential nutrients that support overall well-being.

- **Hydration:** Adequate hydration supports bodily functions, including the absorption of nutrients. Herbal teas, infused water, and nourishing beverages can complement your adaptogen regimen.

- **Micronutrients:** Vitamins and minerals play a crucial role in various physiological processes. Certain adaptogens, like ginseng, might interact with micronutrients, so it's important to maintain balanced levels.

- **Antioxidants:** Antioxidant-rich foods, such as berries, dark leafy greens, and nuts, can enhance the benefits of adaptogens by combating oxidative stress.

- **Adaptogen-Rich Foods:** Some adaptogens can be incorporated directly into your diet. For example, you can add ashwagandha powder to smoothies or brew tulsi tea.

6.2 Sleep and Stress Management

Adaptogens and lifestyle practices that promote stress reduction and restful sleep can work in synergy to enhance your well-being:

- **Stress Management:** Adaptogens are known for their stress-reducing properties, but lifestyle practices like mindfulness, meditation, yoga, and deep breathing can further alleviate stress.

- **Physical Activity:** Regular exercise supports the body's resilience to stress and complements the effects of adaptogens. Aim for a balanced exercise routine that suits your fitness level.

- **Sleep Quality:** Adaptogens like ashwagandha and holy basil can contribute to better sleep quality. Establish a consistent sleep routine, create a calming bedtime environment, and limit screen time before bed.

- **Mindfulness and Relaxation:**
  Incorporate relaxation techniques
  into your daily routine. This can
  include practices like journaling,
  spending time in nature, or
  engaging in hobbies that bring you
  joy.

- **Balancing Work and Rest:**
  Adaptogens can help your body
  adapt to stress, but it's essential to
  create a balance between work,
  rest, and leisure.

Incorporating adaptogens into your
lifestyle is a holistic endeavor that
extends beyond supplementation. By
focusing on a balanced diet, stress
management, and restful sleep, you'll
create an environment where
adaptogens can work in synergy with
your body's natural mechanisms.
Remember that your overall well-
being is the result of the cumulative

effects of various lifestyle factors, including adaptogen use.

6.3 Physical Activity and Exercise

Physical activity and regular exercise play a crucial role in enhancing the effects of adaptogens on your overall well-being:

- **Stress Reduction:** Exercise is a powerful stress reducer. Engaging in physical activity releases endorphins, the body's natural "feel-good" chemicals, which can complement the stress-reducing properties of adaptogens.

- **Cognitive Function:** Physical activity has been linked to improved cognitive function, including memory and mental clarity. This synergy can enhance the cognitive benefits provided by certain adaptogens.

- **Energy and Vitality:** Adaptogens that support energy levels, like ginseng, can work synergistically with exercise to boost overall vitality and endurance.

- **Mood Enhancement:** Regular exercise is known to improve mood and reduce symptoms of anxiety and depression. When combined with adaptogens, this can create a positive cycle of well-being.

6.4 Mindfulness and Meditation

Practicing mindfulness and meditation can amplify the benefits of adaptogens by promoting relaxation, mental clarity, and emotional balance:

- **Stress Reduction:** Mindfulness and meditation techniques, such as deep breathing and progressive muscle relaxation, directly reduce stress hormone levels. When combined with adaptogens, the impact on stress reduction can be more profound.

- **Enhanced Focus:** Adaptogens that support cognitive function, like rhodiola, can work in harmony with mindfulness practices to enhance focus and concentration.

- **Emotional Well-being:** Mindfulness and meditation cultivate emotional awareness and resilience, which aligns with the emotional benefits offered by adaptogens.

- **Sleep Quality:** Mindfulness techniques can improve sleep quality by calming the mind and promoting relaxation. This complements the sleep-enhancing effects of certain adaptogens.

Integrating physical activity, exercise, mindfulness, and meditation into your daily routine can create a comprehensive approach to well-being that synergizes with adaptogen use. These lifestyle practices enhance the effects of adaptogens, creating a holistic strategy for managing stress, improving cognitive function, enhancing mood, and promoting overall vitality. As you embark on this journey, remember that adaptogens and lifestyle factors work together to create a balanced and resilient state of wellness.

CHAPTER 7

Creating an Adaptogenic Wellness Plan

Embarking on a journey of well-being through adaptogens requires careful planning and a personalized approach. we'll guide you through the process of creating an adaptogenic wellness plan that suits your individual needs and goals.

7.1 Personalizing Your Adaptogen Regimen

Designing a personalized adaptogenic wellness plan involves considering your unique health goals, preferences, and lifestyle. Here's how to tailor your regimen:

1. **Identify Your Goals:** Clarify your wellness objectives. Are you seeking stress relief, improved energy, cognitive enhancement, better sleep, or a combination of these benefits?

2. **Research Adaptogens:** Explore different adaptogens and their properties to find the ones that align with your goals. Consider how each adaptogen's effects complement your desired outcomes.

3. **Consult a Healthcare Professional:** Before starting any new supplement regimen, consult with a healthcare provider. They can provide insights based on your

medical history, medications, and individual needs.

4. **Select Your Adaptogens:** Based on your research and professional guidance, choose the adaptogens that best match your goals. You might opt for standalone adaptogens or blends that offer a range of benefits.

5. **Choose the Right Form:** Consider whether you prefer capsules, powders, teas, or other forms. Select a form that aligns with your lifestyle and preferences.

6. **Determine Dosages:** Start with the recommended dosage for each adaptogen and adjust gradually as needed. Take into account any interactions with medications or pre-existing conditions.

7. **Establish a Routine:** Decide when and how you'll incorporate adaptogens into your daily routine. Consider factors like your daily schedule, meal times, and potential interactions with other supplements.

8. **Incorporate Lifestyle Practices:** Integrate stress-reduction strategies, exercise, mindfulness, and sleep hygiene into your routine. These practices synergize with adaptogen use and contribute to holistic well-being.

9. **Monitor and Assess:** Keep a journal to track your adaptogen usage, dosage adjustments, and how you're feeling over time. Monitor your progress and note any changes in your well-being.

10. **Reevaluate Periodically:** Every few weeks or months, reassess your wellness goals and how well your adaptogen regimen is aligning with them. Adjust your plan as needed.

Creating a personalized adaptogenic wellness plan involves thoughtful consideration of your goals, preferences, and health needs. By combining adaptogens with a balanced lifestyle, you can enhance your overall well-being and resilience. Regular communication with a healthcare professional ensures that your plan remains safe and effective. Remember that your adaptogenic journey is a gradual process, and consistent effort will yield the best results over time.

7.2 Tracking Progress and Adjustments

Tracking your progress and making adjustments along the way are essential for optimizing your adaptogenic wellness plan:

1. **Maintain a Journal:** Keep a journal to record your adaptogen usage, dosages, and any changes you observe in your well-being. Note improvements in energy, mood, sleep, and stress levels.

2. **Regular Self-Assessment:** Periodically assess how you're feeling physically, mentally, and emotionally. Compare your current state to when you started your adaptogen regimen.

3. **Wellness Goals:** Revisit your initial wellness goals. Are you experiencing improvements in the areas you wanted to address, such as stress, energy, sleep, or cognitive function?

4. **Dosage and Effects:** Note any changes in your response to the chosen adaptogens. Are you experiencing positive effects, or do you need to adjust dosages for better results?

5. **Lifestyle Factors:** Consider how your lifestyle practices, such as exercise, mindfulness, and sleep, are contributing to your overall well-being alongside adaptogens.

6. **Consult with a Professional:** If you're not experiencing the desired effects or if you're encountering any adverse reactions, consult a

healthcare provider. They can provide guidance on dosage adjustments or alternative adaptogens.

7. **Gradual Changes:** When making adjustments, do so gradually. Incremental changes allow you to assess the effects without overwhelming your system.

8. **Addressing New Goals:** If your goals change or evolve, adjust your adaptogen choices accordingly. For instance, if you initially focused on stress but now want to enhance cognitive function, adapt your plan accordingly.

9. **Stay Informed:** Continue researching and learning about adaptogens. New information might provide insights into better

combinations or dosages for your goals.

10. **Consistency and Patience:** Consistency is key. Adaptogens often yield gradual, cumulative effects. Give your body time to adapt and respond positively.

Tracking your progress and making informed adjustments ensure that your adaptogenic wellness plan remains effective and aligned with your evolving needs. Your journey is unique, and staying attuned to your body's responses is essential. A well-crafted plan, regular communication with healthcare professionals, and the willingness to adapt as you go will lead you toward a more balanced and resilient state of well-being.

7.3 Long-Term Benefits and Sustainable Practices

As you continue to integrate adaptogens into your lifestyle, it's important to consider the long-term benefits and sustainable practices that can enhance your well-being over time.

Adaptogens offer a range of long-term benefits when integrated into a sustainable wellness plan:

1. **Stress Resilience:** Over time, adaptogens can help your body become more resilient to stressors, reducing the impact of chronic stress on your overall health.

2. **Energy Balance:** Consistent use of adaptogens can support balanced energy levels, reducing

the risk of energy crashes or
burnout.

3. **Cognitive Enhancement:** Regular
   consumption of adaptogens that
   enhance cognitive function may
   lead to improved mental clarity,
   focus, and memory over time.

4. **Mood Support:** Adaptogens can
   contribute to a more stable mood
   and emotional well-being as you
   continue to use them.

5. **Sleep Quality:** Integrating sleep-
   supportive adaptogens into your
   routine can lead to sustained
   improvements in sleep quality and
   overall restfulness.

To maintain a sustainable approach to
adaptogen use:

- **Consistency:** Consistency is key
  to experiencing the long-term

benefits of adaptogens. Incorporate them into your routine consistently for optimal results.

- **Variety:** Consider rotating different adaptogens to prevent your body from becoming accustomed to one specific herb. This can maximize their effectiveness over time.

- **Moderation:** While adaptogens can be highly beneficial, avoid over-reliance. A balanced diet, exercise, and other lifestyle factors should also be prioritized.

- **Listen to Your Body:** Pay attention to how your body responds to adaptogens over the long term. Adjust dosages or adaptogen choices as needed based on your evolving needs.

- **Holistic Approach:** Remember that adaptogens are part of a larger wellness picture. Combining them with balanced nutrition, physical activity, mindfulness, and adequate sleep creates a holistic approach to well-being.

- **Regular Check-Ins:** Periodically reassess your wellness goals and how well your adaptogenic plan is meeting them. This ongoing evaluation allows you to refine your approach over time.

- **Professional Guidance:** Maintain open communication with healthcare professionals. Regular check-ins ensure your adaptogen use remains aligned with your health needs and goals.

Integrating adaptogens into a sustainable wellness plan, you're investing in your long-term health and resilience. As you continue on your adaptogenic journey, remember that small, consistent steps can lead to significant improvements over time. Be patient, stay informed, and adapt your approach as needed to create a lasting foundation for well-being.

CHAPTER 8

Recipes and DIY Adaptogen Creations

Incorporating adaptogens into your diet can be both nutritious and delicious. Smoothies are a fantastic way to blend adaptogens with other nourishing ingredients for a well-rounded treat. We will provide you with some adaptogenic smoothie recipes to try.

8.1 Adaptogenic Smoothie Recipes

1. **Berry Bliss Adaptogen Smoothie:**

- Ingredients:

  - 1 cup mixed berries (blueberries, strawberries, raspberries)

  - 1 banana

  - 1 tsp ashwagandha powder

  - 1 tbsp chia seeds

  - 1 cup almond milk (or any milk of your choice)

  - Ice cubes

- Instructions:

  - Blend the mixed berries, banana, ashwagandha powder, chia seeds, and almond milk until smooth.

  - Add ice cubes and blend again until desired consistency is reached.

- Pour into a glass and enjoy this antioxidant-rich and stress-relieving smoothie.

2. **Green Goddess Adaptogen Smoothie:**

- Ingredients:

  - 1 cup spinach leaves

  - 1/2 cucumber

  - 1/2 avocado

  - 1 tsp spirulina powder

  - 1 tsp maca powder

  - 1 cup coconut water

- Instructions:

  - Combine spinach leaves, cucumber, avocado, spirulina powder, maca powder, and coconut water in a blender.

- Blend until creamy and smooth.

- Pour into a glass and savor this green energy-boosting and detoxifying smoothie.

3. **Chocolate-Covered Adaptogen Delight:**

- Ingredients:

  - 1 ripe banana

  - 1 tbsp cacao powder

  - 1 tsp reishi mushroom powder

  - 1 tsp coconut oil

  - 1 cup oat milk (or any milk of your choice)

  - Ice cubes

- Instructions:

  - Blend the ripe banana, cacao powder, reishi mushroom

powder, coconut oil, and oat milk until well combined.

- Add ice cubes and blend again to achieve a creamy consistency.

- Pour into a glass and enjoy this mood-enhancing and immune-supporting chocolate treat.

4. **Tropical Turmeric Adaptogen Smoothie:**

- Ingredients:

  - 1 cup pineapple chunks (fresh or frozen)

  - 1 small mango, peeled and pitted

  - 1 tsp turmeric powder

  - 1/2 tsp ginger powder

  - 1/2 tsp cinnamon powder

- 1 cup coconut water or water

- Ice cubes

- Instructions:

  - Blend pineapple chunks, mango, turmeric powder, ginger powder, cinnamon powder, and coconut water until smooth.

  - Add ice cubes and blend again until desired texture is achieved.

  - Pour into a glass and relish this anti-inflammatory and tropical delight.

Feel free to customize these recipes by adding your favorite fruits, vegetables, and additional superfoods. Remember to start with a lower dosage of adaptogens and gradually adjust as needed. These adaptogenic smoothies can be a delightful and nutritious addition to your wellness routine.

8.2 Herbal Tea Blends

Introduction to Herbal Tea Blends: Herbal tea blends offer a delightful and accessible way to incorporate adaptogens into your daily routine. These blends combine the benefits of adaptogenic herbs with the soothing properties of various other herbs and spices. Here's a deeper look at how to create and enjoy herbal tea blends with adaptogens:

Selecting Adaptogenic Herbs: Begin by choosing the adaptogenic herbs that align with your wellness goals. For example, if you're seeking stress relief, consider ashwagandha or holy basil. If you want to boost energy, opt for rhodiola or ginseng. Combining adaptogens with complementary herbs can enhance both flavor and health benefits.

Pairing Complementary Herbs and Ingredients: To create a balanced herbal tea blend, think about the flavor profiles and health properties of other herbs, spices, and ingredients. For instance:

- **Mint:** Adds a refreshing taste and aids digestion.

- **Chamomile:** Provides a mild, floral flavor and supports relaxation.

- **Lemon Balm:** Offers a citrusy taste and helps reduce stress.

- **Ginger:** Adds warmth and aids in digestion.

- **Turmeric:** Provides an earthy, anti-inflammatory boost.

- **Cinnamon:** Offers warmth and has antioxidant properties.

Creating Your Herbal Tea Blend: Experiment with different combinations of adaptogens and complementary herbs to find a blend that suits your taste buds and wellness needs. Here's a basic recipe to get you started:

1. Start with a base adaptogenic herb like ashwagandha or rhodiola.

2. Add a secondary adaptogen or a complementary herb like mint or chamomile.

3. Include any spices or additional flavorings you prefer, such as

ginger, lemon zest, or
cinnamon.

4. Adjust the quantities to achieve
   your desired flavor and
   strength.

Brewing Herbal Tea Blends:
Brewing herbal tea blends is a simple
process:

1. Boil water and let it cool
   slightly to avoid scalding the
   delicate herbal flavors.

2. Place your herbal blend in a tea
   infuser or a teapot.

3. Pour the hot water over the
   herbs.

4. Allow it to steep for about 5-10
   minutes, or until you reach your
   preferred strength.

5. Remove the herbs or strain the tea to prevent over-steeping, which can make the tea bitter.

Enjoying Your Herbal Tea Blend: Sip your herbal tea blend mindfully. Take a moment to savor the flavors and appreciate the soothing qualities of the herbs. You can enjoy it hot or cold, sweetened or unsweetened, depending on your preferences.

8.3 Incorporating Adaptogens into Meals

Introduction to Incorporating Adaptogens into Meals: While herbal teas are a fantastic way to enjoy adaptogens, you can also incorporate these beneficial herbs into your meals. This approach allows you to diversify your adaptogen consumption and infuse your daily diet with their health-enhancing properties.

Adaptogenic Powders and Tinctures: One of the easiest ways to include adaptogens in meals is by using adaptogenic powders or tinctures. Here's how:

- **Smoothies:** Add a teaspoon of adaptogen powder to your morning smoothie. This pairs well with fruits like berries or bananas and a base of yogurt or plant-based milk.

- **Soups and Stews:** Mix adaptogen tinctures into soups or stews during cooking. This works particularly well with broths, vegetable soups, and slow-cooked dishes.

Incorporating Whole Adaptogenic Ingredients: You can also use whole adaptogenic herbs in your culinary creations:

- **Salads:** Sprinkle dried adaptogenic herbs like astragalus or eleuthero over your salads for an earthy flavor and an immune boost.

- **Stir-Fries:** Incorporate sliced or diced adaptogenic roots like ginseng or maca into stir-fry dishes for added texture and a subtle, nutty taste.

- **Infused Oils and Vinegars:** Create infused oils or vinegars by steeping adaptogenic herbs like ashwagandha or rhodiola in them. Use these for salad dressings or drizzled over roasted vegetables.

Balancing Flavors and Textures: When incorporating adaptogens into meals, consider the overall taste and texture of your dish. Adaptogens often have earthy or bitter flavors, so balance them with other ingredients:

- **Sweet and Savory:** Combining adaptogens with sweet or savory elements can help mask their bitterness. Try adding honey, maple syrup, or savory herbs and spices.

- **Texture:** Experiment with the texture of adaptogens. Grind adaptogenic roots into a powder for a smoother incorporation into dishes.

Start Slow and Monitor Effects: As you begin to incorporate adaptogens into your meals, start with small amounts to assess how your body responds. Monitor your energy levels, stress, and overall well-being to determine the effects of these dietary additions.

Adaptogens are generally safe, but individual reactions may vary. Consult with a healthcare professional if you have specific concerns or health conditions before significantly increasing your adaptogen intake through meals.

Herbal tea blends and incorporating adaptogens into meals offer diverse and enjoyable ways to harness the benefits of adaptogenic herbs in your daily life. Whether you prefer a soothing cup of tea or adding adaptogens to your culinary creations, these methods can enhance your overall well-being when used thoughtfully and in moderation.

www.ingramcontent.com/pod-product-compliance
Lightning Source LLC
Chambersburg PA
CBHW060951260726
48661CB00005B/1844